Maryse Nelson

SECOND TO NONE

"The most successful homecare professional builds an emotionally fulfilling and lucrative career with blocks of compassion, medical competence, excellent judgment and sound business strategies."

Also by Maryse Nelson

From the Ashes

To Haiti with Love

SECOND
TO
NONE

SECOND

TO

NONE

An Essential Orientation and Reference Guide for the Homecare Practitioner

MARYSE NELSON

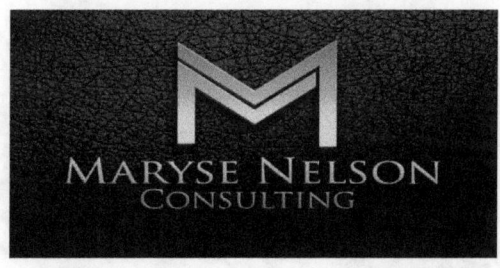

ISBN-10:1540712524
ISBN-13:978-1540712523

I have had the absolute privilege of practicing Physical Therapy for more than two decades in various clinical settings. For many reasons, however, homecare gradually became my passion. The opportunities, rewards and challenges of practicing in the intimate setting of patients' homes, have enabled me to grow professionally while performing my best work. I believe that I have learned more from my patients than I have taught, but I also smile when I think about the many I have been privileged to help. It is that personal satisfaction that has led me to develop this guide as an essential tool for the homecare professional.

This book is dedicated to the entire family of homecare. More specifically, it is for those who see the big picture—those who strive, with every opportunity, to not merely perform the duties of a job, but to help people really live well and overcome the obstacles brought along by disability.

I am grateful to my family and friends for their love and support. I thank Renuka McDavid (Rennie), a great nurse, a friend and a fantastic mentor, along with all the great folks at First Choice Visiting Nurses in Kissimmee, Florida. An equal note of gratitude and professional respect goes to Nurse Minette Williams and Crown Home Care in Kissimmee, Florida.

<u>CONTENTS</u>

INTRODUCTION

This is a guidefor all homecare professionals—the seasoned worker as well as the newcomer. If you are new to homecare, I congratulate you on your achievement.You have gone through the process and are now qualified and ready to join a very distinguished family. You have made a major step and your choice of career places you in the category of special people who want to help improve the lives of others. But before you pick up your bag and supplies and head out to save the world, there are some key elements you need to consider—important tidbitsyou might not have covered in school. Becoming familiar with those points is essential to you becoming successful at both taking care of your patients and ensuring the longevity of your career.

The purpose of this manual is to help you get a strong start in homecare by sharing with you what experience only could have taught me. Starting strong will not only benefit you but also your employer and most importantly, your patients. I am confident that this information, along with the orientation you receive from your agency, will provide the foundation you'll need to start building a successful and rewarding career. You will have plenty of opportunities to learn from your own experience, but for now, keep this guide with you throughout your day. Refer to it often and you will gain the advantage of knowing from the onset, what it took many of us years to figure out. Your journey will be made easier and you will have a better understanding of our business as homecare professionals.

The experienced worker will also find this manual helpful. Although some materials covered will seem familiar, you will find information that will help you fine tune your established system(s) of operation. You will be challenged to consider new, more effective methods of relating to customers and coworkers. My ultimate objective is for the reader to gain a crystal clear understanding of the special union formed by the worker, the patient and the company.When that union is solid, the service that is rendered is second to none.

1 OUR PROFESSION...OUR BUSINESS

The field we are in is very unique. Unlike the supermarket or your favorite clothing store that specializes in selling products, in homecare, we are in the business of selling our *service*. But we also differ from other professionals such as your plumber or your hairdresser who also sell their services. The unique aspect of our profession is that we directly touch our clients—literally and figuratively. We play crucial roles in their fight to survive, to recuperate and to lead more independent, productive lives. We lay our hands on them, we listen to them and we witness their innermost fears. We haveaccess to their personal world, to the most intimate parts of their homes.We are privy to their most sensitive information: their medical record. No one works more closely with these individuals than we do. So not only do we provide a service, but we also have the added responsibility to be more caring, trustworthy and respectful than other workers in the service industry.

Yet, while our profession calls us to be compassionate, we cannot ignore the important fact that we are a business. Sometimes it is very easy to forget that we have a bottom line, that we have deadlines to meet and that, like every other business, we have to be profitable. Although many workers find it very difficult to marry the business principles to thecompassionate facet of homecare, that does not have to be your reality.You simply need to come into this field with a slightly different mentality.

While you trained, I am sure that most, if not all, emphasis was placed on the service delivery aspect of our field. You spent a lot of time learning how to handle patients safely, how to properly administer medications, etc…But in this modern age of brutal competition, that is only one side of the equation. It is important that you view the workforce in its true multidimensional form—that you understand *work* as more than what you individually bring to the table by way of your specialty. In other words, you have to think in a global sense. You are not only a Home Health Aide but you are also a very important team member, responsible as any other worker, for the survival of your company or agency.

So our field is distinctive in the sense that we have to be very careful with the delicate issues surrounding the lives of our patients. Yet, we have to also keep in mind that we have a business to keep afloat.

Now I know what you're thinking: "If I'm a nurse and not an administrator or part of the office staff, why is it my problem to worry about the business side of homecare? Isn't that the job of the owner or the president of the company? Is not my responsibility only to make sure I make my visits and take care of my patients?"

Well, before the world got so competitive and insurance companies became so strict and before patients became so educated, we lived in homecare utopia. We went to work, did our part and everything else was miraculously taken care of for us. But today's world is a lot more demanding—we have to do more and we have to know more to satisfy everyone who has a say in our success. Everyone is held accountable, everyone represents the company. There has never been a more important time than now for workers of any company to function as true team members—for them to clearly understand the importance of everyone's individual duties as well as their collective responsibility and obligation. You can begin to accomplish that goal by becoming very familiar with the mission statement and vision of your company.

Indifference to important business issues relating to work creates inefficiencies or problems that can destroy your company's finances. For example, the simple sin of constantly turning in your notes late delays the billing process which slows down reimbursement, which in turn may increase the time you have to wait for a paycheck. Now that should be important to you because as much as you may love working with people, as much as you may enjoy your patients, I doubt you are in a position financially to not get paid on a regular basis.

Now granted, companies do their very best to pay you on time even when those problems occur. So you may not immediately feel the consequence of your offense. But imagine if you're not the only one and other workers are doing the same. Every second that is spent fixing or trying to deal with that problem is precious time lost—time that is not devoted to acquiring more business or creating lucrative networks or opportunities for the company to prosper.

The work that we do is very rewarding on a humanitarianstandpoint, but it is also our livelihood. At the end of the week, we need it to be converted into food on the table and mortgage payments etc…It is imperative, therefore, that you do everything in your power to be kind but also to have a keen business sense.

After completing the following chapter review questions, let's move into the next sectionwhere you will gain a better understanding of your role as an important team member.

The chapter review questions are designed to stimulate thinking and learning. Greater understanding and better results are achieved when they are discussed in a group setting with a supervisor. If you have tocomplete them on your own,make sure you can comfortably answer every question andIf you need assistance, your supervisor will be more than happy to help!

CHAPTER REVIEW I

1. Why is it important for you to know well your company's mission and vision statements?_____
    _____
    _____
    _____

2. What do we mean by the 'multidimensional' form of homecare?_____
    _____
    _____
    _____

3. Why do you need to understand the many facets of homecare?
    _____
    _____
    _____
    _____

4. How do your actions impact your company's reimbursement rate?_____
    _____
    _____
    _____

5. Keeping in mind technological advances and how fast things change in modern times, name some financial challenges your company may encounter?
    _____
    _____
    _____
    _____
    _____

List, step by step, the billing process of your company. Identify 3 ways you personally could help improve outcome.

_____
_____
_____
_____
_____
_____
_____
_____
_____
_____
_____
_____
_____
_____
_____
_____
_____
_____
_____
_____
_____
_____
_____
_____
_____

2 THE ALMIGHTY REFERRAL

You are hired by a homecare agency and hope there will always be a continuous flow of patients. As you discharge one, in the natural order of things the company should admit one or two new ones. For most of us, this is not a part-time gig. We're in it for the long haul and don't want to see the days that we get sent home or told not to come in at all because the census is low. We are all well aware that in order for each one of us to get paid, the agency has to keep high the demand for its services.

But where do these patients come from and who is responsible for getting them? Whose job is it to ensure that the agency never runs out of patients? The answers to those questions are the main focus of this section. The objective is for you to gain a clear understanding of the referral process and the many ways in which it can be influenced by patients, doctors, homecare workers and administrators alike.

First and foremost, you must understand that competition is fierce out there. For any given geographic area, there are many homecare agencies vying for the same jobs. Doctors' offices and patients have a wide selection of agencies to choose from which means that in order for a company to survive, it not only has to equal its competition, but it has to have a competitive advantage. It has to run its processes smoothly and it has to be effective and efficient. Waste of time, energy, and money has to be at best eliminated and at the very least, kept to a minimum. And all of that has to be done well within legal and ethical guidelines keeping in mind, at all times, the total, complete well-being of our patients.

We're going to go through the referral process in the next few paragraphs. As we do that, try to identify certain areas where your company could or may have a competitive advantage—that is, something it can do better than the competition or something inherent in its practice, location, etc...that gives it an edge over the other companies that serve the same geographic area—somethingthat would make a patient's family or doctor's office choose you instead of the competition.

The referral process most often starts with a Marketer. This is an individual or a firm hired by your agency to generate business or get patients. These workers are responsible for marketing the services of your agency to physicians' offices, hospital discharge planning staff (such as social workers), local community groups/organizations or anyone else who might be in need of a homecare agency. These individuals have to do their work within very strict guidelines imposed by the government. For example, when I first started working, it was common practice for a marketer to reward doctors' offices with gifts as goodwill tokens. Today, there are laws against such practices and violations can result in criminal charges.

When the marketer for your company is out in the field trying to get new patients, he or she comes face to face with marketers from all of the other agencies in your area, or your competition. From that standpoint alone, you can imagine how difficult a task it is to be the chosen one, not taking into consideration several other factors. For example, the person in the office that deals with marketers may like one more than the other or may have more in common with one than the other. An agency may offer a wider variety of services than another(remember competitive advantage?). One agency may be well established in the community with a good track record versus a newer one trying to get its feet wet. You can come up with many other scenarios but the point is that it is not an easy task to accomplish and all workers and owners of homecare agencies should recognize the importance of marketers to the viability and ultimate survival of the company.

So let's say the marketer works really hard and gets one referral. The next order of business is now for the agency staff, once they get the call from the referral source to start their own process. I don't want to get into detailed explanations of what goes on in the office, but generally they deal with all the *t*'s that have to be crossed and the *i*'s that have to be dotted from the standpoint of insurance issues, legal issues, et—allof the technical things that have to be in order before they can actually start calling the field staff to schedule visits for that patient.

Now please take note. Just because I am generalizing the work that takes place in the office, do not underestimate the importance of this process. It is not an easy task. Most times it is very frustrating and the office staff has to concern itself with very vital issues such as reimbursement, deadlines, payroll, etc…They have to coordinate information from the field staff, referral sources, insurance companies, physicians' offices etc...Corporate issues have to be dealt with as well as patients who call in with complaints/concerns and a wide variety of other matters that would take way too much time to go into. During my years of practice, I've come across many field workers who think the office staff just makes copies and calls them with referrals. That train of thought couldn't be farther from the truth. For our purpose here, it is not necessary to delve into every intricacy of office administration, but let me be very clear: if the field staff represents the limbs of the company responsible for delivering the actual service to the patients, then the office staff is the brain that makes vital decisions, relays information, coordinates movements and watches out for everyone.

So now that the referral has been processed by the office and everything checks out, the next step is for it to be passed along to you. You have now received the baton and it is your duty to run the final lap. Your job, regardless of your discipline, is just as crucial to the survival of the company as the job of the marketer and everyone in the office. You are the one who comes face to face with a person, whom until this point, has been nothing but a number or a referral. What you do at the point, the way you care for and treat this individual will be the final action that determines whether the company gets paid or not. Until you have done your part, every work that's gone into this process thus far has been for free. If your part does not materialize, the company has actually lost time and energy, which for a business always translates into money.

So as you receive this referral, in a way, everyone is cheering you on. The marketer, the company and the office staff have all passed their baby down to you and now the spotlight is on you to bring home the bacon. The patient and family members are also eagerly and most times anxiously anticipating your call. As they do, they are hoping that you'll be knowledgeable, that you'll be compassionate and that you'll be considerate. I hope you are beginning to get a sense of how important your role is not only as a caregiver, but also as a business partner. Everything you do once you receive the referral, determines whether or not you and your company will have a gain or a loss.

Complete the chapter review questions, then keep on reading! The next section is all about you, the precious human being who has been entrusted to your care and your agency.

CHAPTER REVIEW II

1. Who in your company is responsible for getting referrals?

    _____

    _____

    _____

2. What exactly do they do to generate a steady flow of patients?

    _____

    _____

    _____

    _____

3. What are some legal guidelines marketers have to follow?

    _____

    _____

    _____

    _____

4. Based on your geographical location, identify your competitors.

    _____

    _____

    _____

    _____

5. Of the ones you identified above, who is your main competitor and why?
    What advantage, if any, do you perceive they may have over your company?

    _____

    _____

    _____

    _____

Within ethical and legal guidelines, list some things you can do individually and as a group to increase your company's competitive advantage.

_____
_____
_____
_____
_____
_____
_____
_____
_____
_____
_____
_____
_____
_____
_____
_____
_____
_____
_____
_____
_____
_____
_____
_____
_____
_____
_____

3

LIFE AFTER THE REFERRAL

So all of the preliminary, expensive work has been done to secure the almighty referral and now it's in your possession. What are the important steps you should take to guarantee success for yourself, your patient and your employer? To make it easier to understand, I have organized the answers to that question into three categories. The following are special tips,information that will help you transition from an average caregiver to a successful homecare professional.

CARINGFOR YOUR PATIENT

For the sake of clarity and a more personal grasp of our subject, let us say that your patient is an adult female by the name of Mrs. Smith. From the very onset, before you even meet her, it is advisable to follow the "golden rule", loosely interpreted as: *treat others like you, yourself, would like to be treated.* Although we hear it often, seldom do we really apply this rule in our lives. You see, the golden rule is part of a set of moral and ethical principles that when followed faithfully, will keep you on the right path both at work and at home. In other words, those principles help improve, prolong and protect all types of relationships and they help keep us out of trouble. So as you meet and begin to work with Mrs. Smith, try to do everything for her as if you were doing it for yourself. With steady practice and experience, you will discover in yourself a more generous and selfless person.

Make Early Contact

Once you receive your referral, as you would appreciate it yourself, call the patient immediately. In homecare, timeliness is everything. There are many important reasons for this but to keep things brief, I'll mention just three. First, it eases the patient's mind. In the ideal situation where the referral is processed quickly, your immediate call will be proof to her that your company is efficient and that she is well thought of. On the other hand, if for any reason there was a delay in the process, your call will have been much awaited and will put an end to the patient's anxious anticipation.

Another reason to call right away is because patients themselves have many appointments to keep and personal affairs to coordinate. Once patients are discharged home, they enter a maze of unfamiliar obligations and personal challenges. The more serious the diagnosis and the less support they have at home, the greater those challenges are. Most patients have to make serious adjustments and modifications to their previous ways of living and time management becomes a very important factor. So an early call from you helps them to navigate their way through the maze with more efficiency and certainty.

The third reason for calling early is that you narrow the window of opportunity for another homecare agency to service the patient. Patients tend to go with whoever calls them first or whoever processes their case faster. Remember, a doctor's order does not give you exclusive rights to the patient. Patients have complete autonomy in choosing an agency and don't ever make the mistake of thinking that you are the only one knocking on their door.

Win the Battle against Lateness

One of the major challenges you will face in the field is that of being on time. It is one of the problems patients complain most about. The nature of our profession, in that context, puts us at a great disadvantage because of all the factors that impact our time. It is not a battle you have to lose, however. The following tips will help you win and keep your patients satisfied.

When you call her to schedule an appointment, don't specify an exact time and explain briefly your reasoning. For example, you don't want to set up a 7:30 appointment but you want to give her your best estimated range (for example, tell her you will arrive between 7:30 and 8:30 although you would do your best to arrive as close to her desired time as possible). You need to consider seriously factors that are not within your control. Traffic, for example, can be your biggest nightmare. Accidents,rubbernecking, bad weather, a funeral procession, roadwork etc…are all enemies to good time management.

Consider also the unpredictable nature of your day to day visits. Although you might have set up a solid schedule, one patient's emergency could derail your entire plans for the day. For instance, a patient who presents with abnormal vital signs or who had a fall during your absence requires a lot more of your time and attention for evaluating and making appropriate contacts. Sometimes you may have to wait for loved ones or paramedics to arrive prior to leaving regardless of your busy schedule.

When such events occur and you cannot help being late, it's imperative that you call the patient at your earliest convenience to inform them. I make a point of informing my patients,on the very first visit, of all the reasons that I could be late to an appointment. I let them know that emergencies are very common in our field and if one should occur with them or any other patient, the problems have to be resolved before I can leave. Educating the patients like this, from the beginning, results in better understanding and acceptance of our occasional shortcomings.

Medicare patientsare required to be homebound in order to qualify for and receive homecare services. It's unfortunate that somehomecare workers make their own interpretation of this rule. In many cases, they use it to make assumptions that the patient should be available to them at any time. They show up to the patient's home whenever they want, sometimes without even the courtesy of a telephone call. As previously stated, we need to respect the patient's time and consider factors in their lives such as other appointments, personal visits, fatigue from sleepless nights, the debilitating impact of pain, long, stressful and difficult morning routines etc…. We really need to be in tune with each patient's world and identify the best way to fit ourselves in it. For the most part, patients are very frustrated and fearful about their medical situations and require our ultimate compassion and consideration. When they sense a disconnect, they know exactly how to fix it: they make a phone call and hire another agency who can better service their needs.

Know Your Profession

Gain the satisfaction of your patient by knowing well your profession and by familiarizing yourself with her case prior to making your visit. Know her history, the reason she went to the hospital in the first place. Know her limitations and use your expertise, in light of that information, to provide the best care you possibly can. Do not ask the patient why she went to the hospital but rather ask her to confirm the reason. That is information you should already have been given. You should have as clear an idea of the patient's journey as you can get. Be prepared, do some research if you have to because patients sense when you don't have a clue about their situation. Don't ever try to "wing it". Prepare for your patient. Consult with the other disciplines on the case to formulate and carry out the best plan of care—one that will help herthe most, in the shortest amount of time.

Continuing education has never been more important than it is today in the world of healthcare. Rules change every day, innovation happens by the second and unless you keep yourself updated in every area of your field, you run the risk of lagging behind and of not effectively servicing your patients.

Keeping yourself up to date does not necessarily have to be a dreadful chore. Your agency goes to great lengths to acquire educational materials both required and suggested. That is your first source of information. Secondly, you are required to fulfill a certain number of continuing education hours for license renewal or recertification. When you take courses, do so to more than satisfy your requirements for renewal. Choose courses that relate to your line of work and will enhance your knowledge and practice. More than anything else, and beyond the need to meet certain criteria for your boss or the government, you owe it to yourself and your patients to self-educate. And that's never been easier than it is today with the help of the internet. The information you seek is readily available and once you start to look into it, you'll be surprised at the speed with which the healthcare world is moving ahead.

Make an attempt to take advantage of as many in-service presentations as possible. The best gift you can give to your patients is sound knowledge of the service you provide. A solid grasp of your specialty is necessary for the patient to make the most progress.

Communication with Other Disciplines is Key

Communicate with the other disciplines treating your patient. In order for you to best care for her, it is essential that everyone seeing Mrs. Smith work toward a common goal. To do that, you have to know what's going on with the patient beyond your field of expertise. For example, I may be seeing a patient for physical therapy but it's important for me to have the nurse's input. Maybe the patient is taking a medication that makes her drowsy at a certain time during the day. It would not be effective for me to schedule a visit during that time. Maybe the patient has a decubitus ulcer that nursing is working really hard to heal but therapy keeps disrupting by having the patient practice bed mobility routines. At times OT and PT may be duplicating services. Sometimes patients admit to social workers noncompliance with nursing or therapy programs. In order to provide the best care to our patients, the right hand has to know what the left hand is doing and the best way to guarantee that is by communicating. A simple telephone call can make all the difference between providing care that is mediocre or good.

Make the patient feel that her health and wellbeing are important to you. When She complainsabout an issue, make sure there is follow through. Do not leave your patient with unresolved conflicts or problems. Whenever you personally are not able to help her, make it your responsibility to communicate her needs to your office or case manager. Refer her to someone who can take care of her.

Respect Your Patient

Respect the patient always. There is a tendency sometimes for healthcare professionals to talk down to certain patients. In body language, speech or mannerism negative messages can easily beconveyed to the patient. Even the most challenging of patients deserve our respect. Never treat your adult patient as you would a child. Even when patients are noncompliant, it is our duty to relate to them firmly, but never in ways that leave them feeling disrespected. A person with limited education can be taught at her own level, but never in a way that is condescending. You will find, as you progress in your career, that certain patients will challenge your value system, your personal preferences, etc…In all cases, it is imperative that they receiveyour very best—even if sometimes your very best is respectfully referring themto another team member who can better serve them.

Respect The Patient's Home

Think about how sacred your home is to you. It is your haven, your safe sanctuary. The same is true for your patient. She, her home and her belongings need to be treated with respect. Be mindful of where you place your articles. Take note, for instance, of her floor and decide whether or not you should remove your shoes.Do not go beyond the point where the patient receives you without informing her and obtaining permission. When performing a home safety evaluation, explain exactly why you need to do it and obtain consent before circulating from room to room. Do not move equipment, furniture or any item from one place to another without returning them to their original position—unless you obtain permission for safety reasons. Handle the patient's home with respect, the same way you would have someone handle yours.

CARING FOR YOURSELF

To care for yourself, in this context, is to know and follow the rules of your profession and your agency; to follow unwritten laws of morality; to motivate yourself to grow and advance; and to do everything in your power to hold on to your license as you treat patients.

Ethics and Professional Responsibility

Let us focus briefly on ethics. The subject of *ethics and professional responsibility* is broader than we could ever do it justice here. For the sake of our discussion, I'll keep things simple by defining it as a set of rules or principles you follow in your profession that lead to right conduct. It deals with the rightness and wrongness of actions or behaviors. At the very core of those principles is the concept of morality. I'm sure you can think of some people that naturally seem to be highly ethical and others who come up short.

You make ethical decisions every day both in your personal and professional life. I advise you to make every effort to keep your ethical standards as high as possible. If you find yourself struggling in any area, consider the behavior or action and ask yourself the following questions:

1. *How would I feel if my family knew I was doing this?*
2. *Is my action or behavior legal?*
3. *How would I feel if my picture and action made first page in the morning newspaper? Would I feel proud?*

If you cannot answer in the positive for any one of those three questions, seriously rethink your move. You can save yourself a world of shame and professional trouble by paying close attention to your actions and making sure you operate well within your profession's ethical boundaries.

Communication and Documentation

In our profession, you care for yourself with your communication and documentation (they are not two different concepts—documentation is a form of communication—however, for the sake of clarity here, let's treat them as such). You can NEVER communicate too much. It is essential on every single level and in every form. I am sure your company has gone over the necessity of proper communication and documentation to ensure optimal patient care, to facilitate cohesiveness among the disciplines, to guarantee reimbursement and to protect employees and the company from a legal standpoint. I cannot emphasize enough the importance of this subject. Here are some tips that will help you:

a. *Enter information in the patient's log (found in the folder you keep in their home) every time you make a visit. Although every company's log may vary slightly in content, it generally asks for the patient's vital signs, a brief explanation of your treatment, and anything else you want communicated to the other disciplines treating the patient. Every time a page of the log is completed, it should be the responsibility of the person making the last entry to turn the original copy in to their agency. Those original copies could potentially help you in the courtroom one day.*

b. *What you find out during your visits or what the patients tell you are not for you alone. Remember, it takes a team of professionals to provide the best care to our patients. If my patient's vital signs are abnormal, I report it to the doctor's office, the case manager, and the folks that run the show at the office. Anything unusual with my patient gets reported to somebody. For instance, any new medical complaints or findings, missed visits, if the patient refuses care, if the patient is requesting new services, etc…it all gets reported.Now having said that, as you gain experience you'll get better at determining what to report and to whom. You don't want to be calling physicians' offices with every minor complaint.However, what may seem minor to you sometimes could be a big deal to the doctor—that's where your supervisors come in. Never feel like you're bothering them with your phone calls. They want to know what's going on out in the field. So at the very least, if you're a little unsure about calling the doctors sometimes, then call the case manager or supervisor at the office and get their advice. **Note: Confidentiality guidelines are honored here as information is being shared only with people who are involved in the patient's care.***

c. *ALWAYS follow your oral communication with written documentation. Every phone call you make, every report you give, every time you discuss something important with your patients, doctors, family members or anyone else, it is absolutely essential that you either include it in your visit note or write a separate communication note altogether. This written document is the only proof you have of that interaction. Be very diligent when it comes to translating your oral discussions into solid, written reports.*

When you communicate and document effectively, you not only protect your patient's best interest, but you also protect yourself legally. I recently watched a nationally televised court case in which the expert witness, a doctor, was being grilled on treatment he rendered a year ago. The good doctor relied very heavily on his notes and he stated many times that it was impossible to remember every detail of what he did a year ago.

In our profession, workers often find themselves testifying in court. Attempting to rely solely on your memory would not only be unprofessional, it would be virtuallyimpossible given the number of patients we treat every day—and very often, the proof is in the details which we tend to easily forget about. So communicate and document as if your life depends on it. Oneday, it just might.

CARING FOR YOUR COMPANY

By now I hope you realize that you, the patient and the company are inextricably linked. It is a three way partnership or relationship where each entity depends on the othersand the tighter the bonds among the three, the stronger the unit. Please note that in caring for the patient, you automatically benefit yourself and the company. In caring for yourself, you automatically benefit the patient and the company. In caring for the company, you automatically benefit the patient and yourself. For example, let's examine the subject of knowing well your profession. If you take that advice you will reach your primary goal of providing the best care to your patient. But also note that you will also increase your knowledge base and willbe less likely to make costly errors (benefit to you, benefit to company). Think of all the problems you'll avoid by not making those errors. You also increase your value in the marketplace—you become a great commodity. Your company will be respected and viewed as having competent, knowledgeable workers (benefit to company). A competent, knowledgeable team is a *competitive advantage* which means the patient is more likely to call back with future needs and also *refer*others to your agency. This is the best kind of referral your company could hope for—one that comes virtually free of charge.

Patients do not keep quiet. They tell their doctors, friends and family members all about the quality of care they receive from healthcare agencies. It's in your best interest to make sure those reports are positive. Remember, when you do things right, the entire team wins. The opposite also holds true.

Let's now look at some business principles you can use to further benefit your company:

Market Continuously

"*Are you kidding me? I'm not a Marketer!*" That might be your initial thought but indeed you are. As you care for patients, as you fine tune your skills, as you communicate with people in your field, you are either marketing or making yourself more *marketable*. The clothes that you wear to work, the way you carry yourself, your attitude, and your willingness (or unwillingness) to help people are all commercials you are producing. That is the reason it is very important to be ethical and to make every effort, in all things, to stay in the positive realm.

In modern times we say a video, for example, has gone viral when it becomes very popular due to sharing on the internet via email, the social media websites, etc…The idea is based on the way an actual virus attacks the cells of the human body. They get in, replicate themselves many times over and very quickly cause one cell to infect all others around it. It is the job of every cell that becomes infected to pass the virus along to everyone in its world.

This brings us to the concept of *viral marketing*. It is a form of advertising that gets people to spread a particular message and it has been proven to be more effective than its non-viral counterparts. In viral marketing, a person passes on information to everyone in their world and all those people do the very same thing. In a very short period of time, you can understand how fast that information can circulate and the icing on the cake is the *validity* of the message. Everyone receives it from someone they know. It's a testimony from a trusted source. Viral marketing is the old fashioned "word of mouth" strategy, exponentially increased due to modern technology.

So what does all this mean for you? Am I asking you to launch marketing campaigns? Not at all, but if you understand the basic concepts you will become an automatic advertising machine. Doing everything we've discussed in this chapter already puts you in that position. When your patient receives great care, she becomes viral in spreading your professionalism, your compassion and your company name to everyone in her world. So without really emphasizing the subject, you have actually created a marketer in that patient. Do your work in a way that makes every patient you treat go viral!

Other Customers to Consider

Because your agency is also your business, consider every one of their customers as your very own. Every one of those customers could potentially affect your pocket book. But who are those customers? Very simple: your patients are primary but your customers also include the medical equipment companies, the doctor's offices, the insurance companies, in fact, everyone who has or can potentially have a stake in your business. So everyone you come in contact with who has something to gain or lose from your business is a customer. Doing your best to have a winning attitude and keeping all your customers happy is great marketing strategy that directly benefits your company. Think of each customer as a functional networkrather than an individual. In doing so, you will better appreciate each customer's real value to your company.

Relating To Team Members

Do yourself, your company and your patients a huge favor and respect every discipline on your team. Recognize everyone's individual specialty as being important and steer clear of people's toes. Communicate with respect and understanding. Do not criticize one coworker with another and absolutely never, with a patient. Instead, help that person become better by being truthful in a respectable manner. Know how to deliver bitter pills—provide a soothing balm whenever necessary. Highlight someone's accomplishments instead of being jealous. Pass along compliments from patients and their families—everyone needs to be encouraged, everyone likes to be validated. Don't be the person who always throws stones but never has a kind word to share. Picture all the other disciplines, the office staff and the administrators above you as one team—each member performing a different function, but all working toward the same goals of keeping patients healthy, keeping customers happy, keeping the business afloat and keeping food on the table for a long time to come.

CHAPTER REVIEW III

1. Discuss in detail the ethical issues that workers in your company may struggle with. What are the consequences of making poor decisions relating to those issues?

    _____

    _____

    _____

    _____

2. Discuss as a group the specific methods your company could use to begin 'viral marketing'?

    _____

    _____

    _____

    _____

3. List 5 things you, as an individual worker, can do to increase patient volume:

    _____

    _____

    _____

    _____

4. Name 3 reasons documentation and communication are so important in your line of work.

    _____

    _____

    _____

    _____

5. Who are your customers? List as many as possible:

    _____

    _____

    _____

    _____

What habits could your company develop to satisfy as many of those customers as possible?

_____
_____
_____
_____
_____
_____
_____
_____
_____
_____
_____
_____
_____
_____
_____
_____
_____
_____
_____
_____
_____
_____
_____
_____
_____

AFTERWORD

I would like to thank you for devoting precious time to learn more about the business we're in.Good solid advice goes a long way in the field of homecare, so do your best to follow the recommendations in this manual with great care. Remember:

- *The patient is key—aim to always satisfy.*
- *Be proactive and anticipate needs before they arise.*
- *Communicate effectively to prevent mole hills from becoming mountains.*
- *Treat every co-worker as a vital part of the team.*
- *Empower your co-worker by advising with respect and make it a habit to provide positive reinforcement.*
- *Report, always, to your supervisors.*
- *Become a marketing machine with your attitude, professionalism and creativity.*
- *YOUR PROFESSIONAL SURVIVAL DEPENDS ENTIRELY ON THE WAY YOU TREAT YOURSELF, YOUR PATIENT AND YOUR AGENCY.*

The homecare profession extends far beyond a routine occupation. It requires responsibility, commitment, compassion, professionalism, strong ethical values, good business sense and a lot of loveas foundation and fuel. In this field, every body you wash, every medication you dispense, every exercise program you instruct, every fall you help prevent, every articulation of words you facilitate, every social program you coordinate and every caregiver you encourage, is a great contribution to humanity.Continue to build a wonderful professional legacy—Sign your work with excellence!

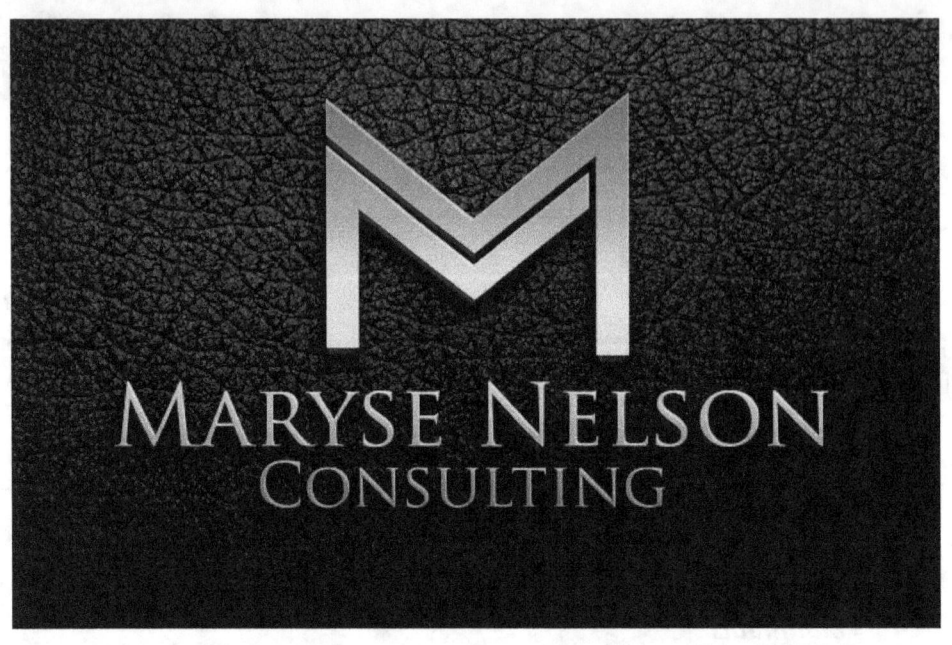

HEALTH…BUSINESS…COMPASSION

Always Reaching Higher!

TEACHING, TRAINING AND PROBLEM-SOLVING

407-346-1590

MARYSE@CONSULTNELSON.COM

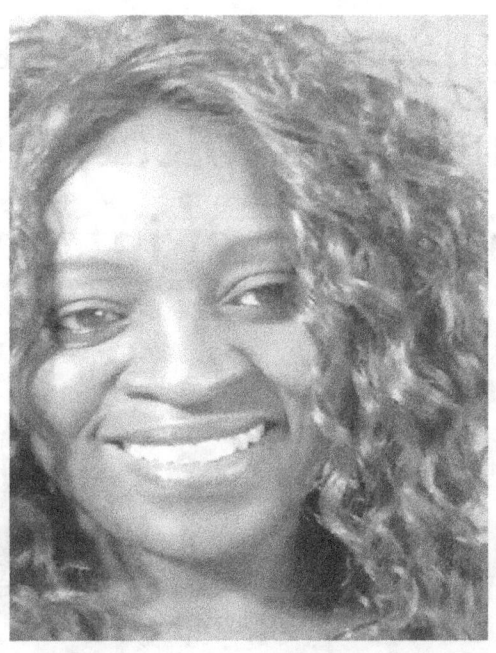

Maryse Nelson is the founder and president of Samarita Ministries, Inc. and MARYSE NELSON CONSULTING. She enjoys motivating and empowering individuals to attain higher standards in life via seminars, conferences, private sessions and written material. Maryse is a physical therapist of many years and also holds an MBA degree. She travels throughout the United States training in the areas of health and business with an emphasis on the importance of compassion. When not working, Maryse enjoys reading, writing, spiritual retreats and spending quality time with her family in Kissimmee, Florida.

To order copies of this guide or schedule on-site seminars or presentations, please use the following contact information:

MARYSE NELSON CONSULTING

Maryse Nelson

Phone: 407-346-1590
Fax: 407-930-9012
E-mail: maryse@consultnelson.com

Our books are also available at amazon.com.

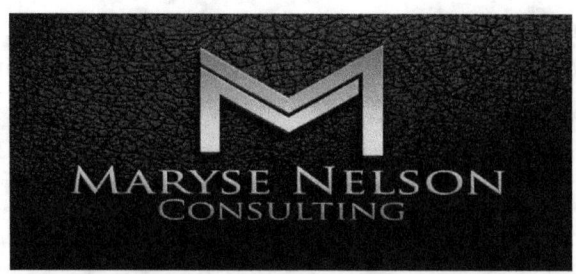

www.ingramcontent.com/pod-product-compliance
Lightning Source LLC
Chambersburg PA
CBHW081306180526
45170CB00007B/2588